YOUR KNOWLEDGE HAS VALUE

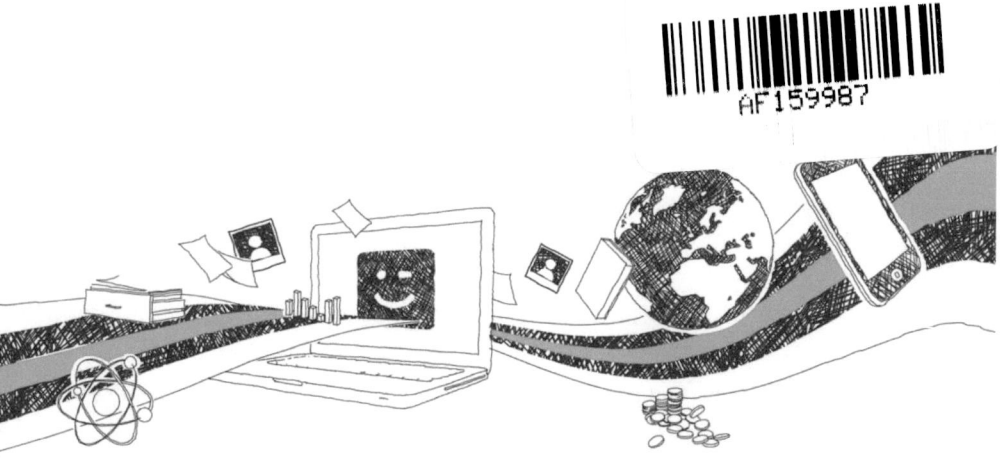

- We will publish your bachelor's and master's thesis, essays and papers

- Your own eBook and book - sold worldwide in all relevant shops

- Earn money with each sale

Upload your text at www.GRIN.com
and publish for free

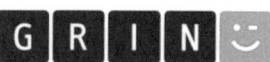

Bibliographic information published by the German National Library:

The German National Library lists this publication in the National Bibliography; detailed bibliographic data are available on the Internet at http://dnb.dnb.de .

This book is copyright material and must not be copied, reproduced, transferred, distributed, leased, licensed or publicly performed or used in any way except as specifically permitted in writing by the publishers, as allowed under the terms and conditions under which it was purchased or as strictly permitted by applicable copyright law. Any unauthorized distribution or use of this text may be a direct infringement of the author s and publisher s rights and those responsible may be liable in law accordingly.

Imprint:

Copyright © 2015 GRIN Verlag, Open Publishing GmbH
Print and binding: Books on Demand GmbH, Norderstedt Germany
ISBN: 978-3-668-03754-0

This book at GRIN:

http://www.grin.com/en/e-book/305672/no-woman-should-die-while-giving-birth-a-discussion-on-the-progress

Leonard Kabongo

"No Woman Should Die While Giving Birth". A Discussion on the Progress Made and Limitations on Achieving the MDG5 in Namibia

GRIN Publishing

GRIN - Your knowledge has value

Since its foundation in 1998, GRIN has specialized in publishing academic texts by students, college teachers and other academics as e-book and printed book. The website www.grin.com is an ideal platform for presenting term papers, final papers, scientific essays, dissertations and specialist books.

Visit us on the internet:

http://www.grin.com/

http://www.facebook.com/grincom

http://www.twitter.com/grin_com

TITLE: "NO WOMAN SHOULD DIE WHILE GIVING BIRTH": A DISCUSSION ON THE PROGRESS MADE AND ONGOING LIMITATIONS IN ACHIEVING THE MILLENNIUM DEVELOPMENT GOAL 5 IN NAMIBIA.

Table of contents

1 Introduction 3

2 Background to the Millennium Development Goals agenda 4

3 Background to the Namibian Health Status 5

4 Programs and policies developed for the attainment of MDG5 in Namibia 6

5 Way forward 8

References 9

1 Introduction

The fifth Millennium Development Goal (MDG5) calls for improving maternal health and focuses on two specific objectives: the reduction of global maternal mortality ratio (MMR) by two third and the universal access to reproductive health by the year 2015 (United Nations, 2013).

Recent data shows that globally the Maternal Mortality Ratio has seen a significant decrease from 400 per 100,000 live births in 1990 to 260 per 100,000 live births in 2008 (Zere et al, 2011). Despite this world progress, some 300,000 women died in 2013 from causes related to pregnancy and childbirth whereby 62% of the deaths occurring in Sub-Saharan Africa (United Nations, 2014).

Access to a comprehensive package of reproductive health services has seen an improvement with 83% of pregnant women attended by a skilled health worker at least once during their pregnancy in 2012 compare to 65% in 1990 (United Nations, 2014).

According to the United Nations (2014), there remain extreme differences in maternal mortality among countries with almost one third of global deaths concentrated in India (17%) and Nigeria (14%); with Sierra Leone being the Country with the highest MMR (1100 per 100,000 live births) while Belarus has the lowest (1 per 100,000 live births).

Namibia is one of the affected sub-Saharan countries. It is estimated that, everyday a woman dies in Namibia due to complications related to either pregnancy or childbirth. The Maternal Mortality ratio has increased from 225 per 100,000 live births in 1992 to 271 per 100,000 live births in 2000 and 449 per 100,000 live births in 2007/2008 (WHO, 2009).

This data has put the Country on a balance scale to initiate and develop policies and programs for the acceleration of the reduction of MMR against set targets and reverse the trends to achieve 75% reduction in accordance with the MDG5 target.

The purpose of this paper is to critically analyze policies, strategies and programs that were developed in Namibia to meet the global and country targets for the attainment of the MDG5. Also to evaluate the progress made, discuss challenges and identify way forwards for local and global response.

This essay will review the Millennium Development Goals agenda, the Namibian Country health status in the context of MDG 5 and the policies, strategies and programs developed to mitigate Maternal Mortality and access to comprehensive sexual and reproductive health services. A discussion on progress made and limitations experienced will pave the way forwards to the local and global response to achieve this most important goal.

2   Background to the Millennium Development Goals agenda

In September 2000 a total number of 189 United Nations General Assembly member states adopted the Millennium Declaration (MD) after which eight smart, measurable, achievable, realistic goals/targets were developed - the Millennium Development Goals (MDGs) that are implemented by developing Countries with assistance from their developed member Countries (NPC,2013). The eight MDGs are

MDG1: Eradicate extreme poverty and hunger

MDG2: Achieve universal primary education

MDG3: Promote gender equality and empower women

MDG4: Reduce child mortality

MDG5: Improve maternal health

MDG6: Combat HIV/AIDS, malaria and other diseases.

MDG7: Ensure environmental sustainability

MDG8: Develop a global partnership for development.

A particular emphasis has been put on health related MDGs (4, 5, &6) because of the essence they carry for the global sustainable development. Every individual irrespective of their race, age, sex has a right to good health and well-being. A mentally and physically stable Nation will enhance economic growth and prosperity.

In this paper I draw attention on Namibia, a very interesting and complex Country that has incorporated the health related MDGs in the National Policy Frameworks for Social and Economic Development (WHO and MOHSS, 2010).

3 Background to the Namibian Health Status

Namibia is situated in the Southwest part of Africa covering an area of 824,000km^2. The country population is 2, 1 million with an annual growth rate estimated at 2.5 with sparsely population of which the majority live in the six Northern Regions where the density is higher than the national average of 2.2 per square meter.

Namibia is classified as upper middle income Country however the most inequal society in the World (MOHSS and WHO, 2010). Despite the small population, the Health and Demographic Survey conducted in 2007 indicates that the Country experiences critical socio-economic and health challenges that pose a threat to his national development plan agenda. In 2008, the employment rate was estimated at 37%, third of the population was estimated to be poor with 34% only having access to sanitation (NDHS, 2007).The health system inherited from the Colonial Government remained fragmented with services concentrated in the urban areas .The Ministry of Health and Social Services is the custodian of the Namibian health and wellbeing. Its mandate is to deliver quality health care services to the Namibian people. The Ministry operates in 9 National Directorates and 13 Regional Directorates. Primary Health care is the guiding principle for health care delivery in the Country. Health services are organized from outreach points (1,150), Clinics and Health posts (285), Health centers (30), District Hospitals (34), Intermediate Hospitals (3) to National referral Hospital (1).

According to the same survey (NDHS, 2007) ,Maternal Mortality Ratio has doubled from 249 per 100,000 live births in 1992 to 449 per 100,000 live births in 2000 despite the increased in Skilled Birth attendance (80%) and Antenatal care coverage (95%).

This pick was attributed to the high HIV prevalence rate (18%) among pregnant women as an indirect cause and to direct major causes including hypertension disorders, obstructed labour, haemorrhage and post-partum sepsis. All of them being preventable causes, the Ministry of Health and Social Services in Namibia together with development partners WHO and European Union have developed programs and strategies to reduce the trend of MMR from 449 per 100,000 live births to 50 per 100,000 live births and achieve the MDG5 by 2015. In 2010, Namibia reported a Maternal Mortality Ratio of 200 per 100,000 live births, an infant mortality rate of 46 per 1000 live births and child mortality of 69 per 1000 live births (CIA, 2014; UNICEF, 2010). The skilled birth attendance is reported at 95% (target achieved?) while universal access to reproductive health shows little progress. The contraceptive prevalence rate stands at 46.6% (MDG target 100%) and Teenage pregnancy at 15% (MDG target 0%) (UNDP, 2012).

At this trend, there is need for drastic reduction of MMR in Namibia and improvement of access to reproductive health services to achieve the MDG5 set targets.

Programs and strategies were developed for this purpose.

The progress made, challenges and limitations in these programs are discussed in the following section.

4 Programs and policies developed for the attainment of MDG5 in Namibia

During the launching of the PARMMA in Namibia, the Minister of Health and Social Services in his speech said: "No woman should die while giving birth" (WHO, 2009). The Namibian Government is committed to achieve the Millennium Development Goals as this aspiration is shown in the country's vision 2030: "*A prosperous and industrialized Namibia, developed by her human resources, enjoying peace, harmony and political stability.*"(NPC, 2004).Under this umbrella, multi-sectoral projects were developed to meet the national targets in line with the MDGs. The Ministry of Health and Social Services in Namibia has launched various programs, strategies and Policies to address the MDG 5 challenges. In 2009, Namibia joined the rest of Africa by launching the ''Campaign on Accelerated Reduction of Maternal Mortality in Africa'' (CARMMA) followed in 2013 by the Programme for the Acceleration of the Reduction of Maternal and Child Mortality (PARMaCM).

These programs support a road map for implementation to address challenges to the MDG5.The multi-sectoral structures put in place focus on the reduction of the 3 delays identified as contributing factors to maternal death: delay in seeking help, accessing health institution and receiving appropriate health care (WHO, 2009).

Other interventions included training of trainers on life saving skills and Emergency Obstetric Care ,improve referral systems, conduct routine reviews of maternal deaths, improve procurement and infrastructure, avail essential medicine to rural areas, strengthen adolescent and sexual reproductive health and improve access to PMTCT services across the Country (UNDP, 2012).

In the recent Namibian Demographic and Health Survey (NDHS, 2013), key findings show that there hasn't been enough progress made to meet the MDG target. The MMR is 385 per 100,000 live births in 2013 while the target is 50 per 100,000 live births. Actually MMR has increase from 2000 although the survey explains that the difference in increase is not statistically significant. This indicates that Namibia is unlike to achieve the MDG5 targets. See figure below.

Maternal Mortality ratio trends-Namibia

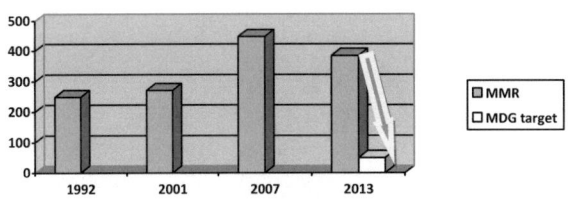

When assessing access to comprehensive reproductive health, the same survey showed that the use of contraceptives has increased from 37% in 2000 to 50% in 2013. However the use of a modern method is 53 percent among women in the highest wealth quintile versus 39 percent among women in the lowest wealth quintile. (NDHS, 2013). Ninety-seven percent (97%) of women received antenatal care from a skilled provider with 87% of institutional deliveries whereby 88% where attended by a skilled provider. This is interesting result since skilled attendance at delivery is been promoted in Developing Countries to address the high Maternal/Perinatal morbidity and mortality (Nyango D.et al, 2010).

However, only 73 percent of births to women in the lowest wealth quintile were delivered by a skilled provider, in contrast to 98 percent of births to women in the highest quintile (NDHS, 2013).This shows inequities in the access to maternal health care services. A few years ago, Zere et al (2010) pointed out that women in Namibia urban areas are delivered by skilled providers 30% more than their rural counterpart and challenged that the rich use public health facilities 30% more than the poor.

In the Survey (NDHS, 2013), 28% of women report that getting money for treatment is a serious concern to access care when sick and 31% indicate that distance to the health facility is a problem.

The issue of inequality and inaccessibility to health care services could be at the centre of the Namibian Health System and a major constraint to achieve the MDG5. Other challenges include shortage of skilled health workers especially in rural areas, high staff attrition rate, non availability of essential drugs in rural areas, inadequate community outreach slow implementation of decentralization and poor record keeping, monitoring and evaluation. In this context, what should be the local and global response?

5 Way forward

Locally there is need to refine Policies and plans addressing the MDG 5 beyond 2015 especially that now the Namibia Demographic and Health survey has been released. In the context of inequities, it's difficult to reduce the maternal mortality ratio and achieve the MDG5 because a large segment of the population has limited access to essential obstetric care and basic social services. This approach should be multisectoral involving all stakeholders to address the social determinant of health in line with the recommendations of the Commission on Social Determinant for Health and the Primary Health Care. Namibia should develop staff training programs and strategies for retention in public sector in a Country where 60% of Doctors practice in the private sector (WHO and MOHSS, 2010).

Globally, there is need to develop a system of accountability through the support of quality and sustainable data to ensure that resources are allocated where needed. Looking beyond the MDG era, the international agencies should support Countries efforts to build on progress made. Requejo and the countdown 2015 writing team (2014) support that massive inequalities in intervention coverage and health outcomes must be tackled for progress to continue. Countries must share their experiences in achievement of MDGs. Countries should strengthen training of midwives and midwifes leaders to drive future strategies and influence health outcomes. Maternal death reduction will require a health system solution. All stakeholders, Non Governmental Organizations, State agencies, civil societies and the community at large should be actively involved for a pregnant woman to meet with the right person, at the right place and at the right time.

References

Central Intelligence Agency (2014).The word factbook. Maternal Mortality rate. [Online] available at www.cia.gov

National Planning Commission (2004). National Plans. Vision 2030. Windhoek. Namibia. [Online] .Available at www.npc.gov.na

National Planning Commission (2013). Millennium Development Goals. Progress report number 4.windhoek.Namibia

Nyango D., Mutihir J., Laabes E., Kigbu J.,Buba M.,(2010).Skilled attendance: The Key Challenges to Progress in Achieving MDG5 in North Central Nigeria. *African Journal of Reproductive Health. June 2010,* 14 (2) pp 129

Requejo J.H. et al (2014). Countdown to 2015 and beyond: fulfilling the health agenda for women and children. *The Lancet Volume 385,* No 9966, page 466-476.

The Namibia Ministry of Health and Social Services (MoHSS) and ICF International (2014). The Namibia Demographic and Health Survey 2013. Windhoek, Namibia, and Rockville, Maryland, USA: MoHSS and ICF International.

The Namibian Ministry of Health and Social Services (2007). Namibia Demographic and Health Survey 2006/2007.Windhoek.Namibia.

UNICEF (2010).Working Toward Development. [Online] access at http://www.unicef.org/namibia/overview_13592.html

United Nations (2014). Millennium Development Goals Report 2014.New York 2014

United Nations Development Programme (2012).Improve Maternal Health. [Online] available at http://www.in.undp.org/content/namibia/en/home/mdgoverview/overview/mdg5. html

United Nations, UNDP, UNFPA, UNICEF (2013).The Millennium Development Goals Report 2013.[Online] available at http://www.un.org/millenniumgoals/beyond2015-news.shtml

WHO (2009). Namibia steps Up against Maternal Mortality. News Break. Maternal health. Issue 3, page 4 [Online] available at www.afro.who.int/.../4266-newsbreak-maternal-health-issue-3-december.

WHO and MOHSS (2010). Namibia Country Cooperation Strategy 2010-2015. Abridged version. Windhoek. Namibia

Zere, E. Oluwole, D. Kirigia, J.M. Mwikisa, C.N. and Mbeeli, T. (2011). Inequities in skilled attendance at birth in Namibia: A decomposition analysis, *BMC Pregnancy and Childbirth,* 11(34) *doi:* 10.1186/1471-2393-11-34

YOUR KNOWLEDGE HAS VALUE

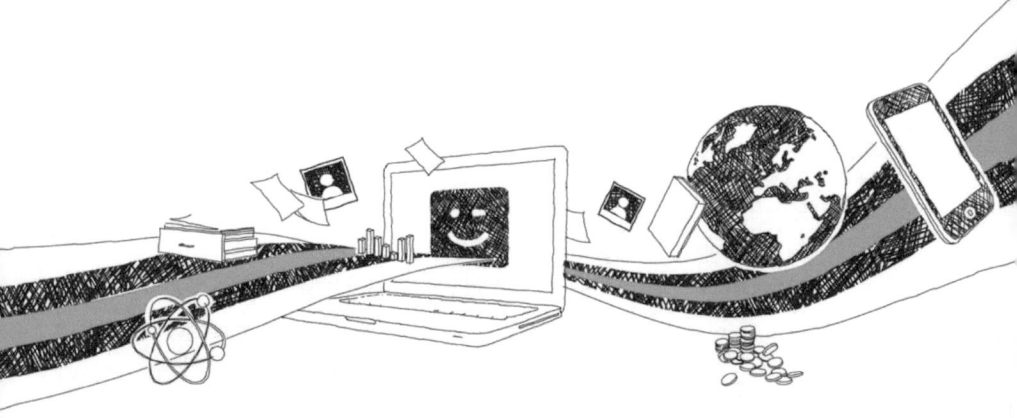

- We will publish your bachelor's and master's thesis, essays and papers

- Your own eBook and book - sold worldwide in all relevant shops

- Earn money with each sale

Upload your text at www.GRIN.com
and publish for free

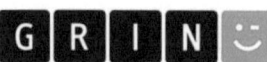